Table of Contents

A Key The Books of Ainslie Meares. Synopses of 33 books.
By Owen Bruhn. Author & Publisher.
  ISBN 978-0-6481084-1-2
  Cover and graphic design. Sarah Bruhn

Dedication

After Ainslie Meares' passing his Estate published several manuscripts that would otherwise never have seen the light of day. They boosted the number of his books in circulation. Their work deserves wider acknowledgement. This "Key" aims to supplement it.

The first line index from The Silver Years inspired indexing the rest of Ainslie Meares' poetry books.

Pauline McKinnon has kept Ainslie Meares' torch alight creating and training a network of teachers; something Meares' was unable to do before his unexpected passing. This little book would most likely not have been written but for her work and example.

Disclaimer

This book is intended for general information only. It should not be used as a substitute for consulting a qualified health practitioner. Neither the author nor the publisher can accept any responsibilty for your health or any side effects of methods in this book or books cited herein.

Copyright

Finding and Buying Meares' Books

Finding Them

Ainslie Meares' books can be sourced through the internet, second hand book sellers and some libraries.

If you are lucky you might be able to look at a copy of one or two of Meares' books at your library. Unfortunately, the stocks in libraries tend to be depleted as the books have been loaned for decades, wear out and are withdrawn from the shelves.

Libraries don't purchase second hand books. If library access happens to be your only option then you could ask the library to order a book about Meares' method written by other authors (see p44).

After the library, you could look into second hand book sellers or the internet. This "Key" book was prepared so people can preview Meares' books before finding and buying them from these sources. It has short synopses of 33 to help decide which one to get.

Buying Them

Obviously, people would like cost estimates for each book. These are impossible to provide as the prices vary and depend on:

- The individual book.
- Condition. "New" book is an exageration made by some suppliers as Meares' books are only available second hand. "New" really means excellent condition. Books in good or average condition generally sell for less.
- Hard cover generally costs more than soft cover.
- Most of the books advertised have no jacket.
- Autographed copies cost more.
- Postage may be included or may be extra. Some suppliers charge high postage fees (don't get caught out).
- Currency. The same number may cost more if it is not your currency (eg UK Pounds vs USD vs Euro vs AUD).

In 2016, an extensive search indicated that several of Ainslie Meares' 35 books were hard to source. That number may increase over time.

This "Key" book provides you short synopses and the length of 33 books. This will also help determine the value of the subject matter in each book to you, the reader.

This Key also includes a short biography of Ainslie Meares. Knowing a little about him will also help your choice. For example, publication dates may be compared with dates of the Hypnosis, Relief Without Drugs and Stillness Meditation Periods.

Non-Fiction Books (21)

This book has synopses of 21 of Meares' non-fiction books. Each synopses is similar to a table of contents with 8-24 points, each point being 1-3 lines in length (up to 10 lines for some "technical" books). In 2 cases the synopses is a brief description.

Works Of Fiction (2)

Synopses would be of little assistance and aren't provided for:
1. The Kiss of Jocasta (A play)
2. Where Magic Lies - A story about life with almost poetic overtones as only Ainslie Meares would write it.

Poetry Books (12)

This Key has first line indexes for all Meares' 12 poetry books. Choosing a book using the first line index doesn't need a lot of precision. A sense that several first lines look interesting will suffice.

Meares explains in his writings that he wrote poetry, during the Stillness Meditation, as a "tool" to help learn his style of meditation.

How Distant The Stars was written early in the Hypnosis Period well before Meares had transitioned to teaching meditation. Most likely, How Distant The Stars, won't help you learn how to meditate. One or more of the later poetry books are a better choice.

If you decide that viewing some samples would help confirm your choice might consider accessing Ainslie Meares on Meditation. That book includes 30 of Ainslie Meares' poems, a couple from each poetry book (also see p44). How the poetry fits in is also explained in that book.

Miscellaneous

A list of Ainslie Meares' braille, audio and translated books is provided. The book finishes with a list of books and CDs by other authors about Meares' method.

About Ainslie Meares (1910-1986)

Ainslie Meares was the son of a gentleman doctor and had a sheltered upbringing. He decided to become a farmer, studied agriculture and then went on to study medicine. He joined the army and became involved in psychiatry towards the end of World War 2.

Hypnosis Period (before ~1960)
He became one of several psychiatrists using hypnosis as an uncovering technique. He was able to hypnotise his patients so deep they could hardly talk, so he showed them how to draw. Some could not hold a pencil, but they could model clay. In turn, they were able to show him the hidden depths of the human mind.

Meares decided that it was being hypnotised rather than the treatments that went with it that benefited his patients. He came to believe that the state of hypnosis was a temporary step back to a simpler restorative state of mind. If this step back did not occur at regular intervals then there could be a build up of anxiety and hurtful pain due to lack of mental rest.

Relief Without Drugs Period (~1960-1970)
In 1960 Meares was elected President of the International Society of Hypnosis. By then he had transitioned from hypnosis to meditation. In hypnosis, he was active and the patient passive. In meditation, he showed patients how to do it all themselves. The ultimate state of mind being very similar. In the 1950s Meares had helped many people learn to relieve pain (especially from cancer). Meares travelled to Asia to meet mystics said to be able to control pain. Eventually, he met an old yogi who he talked with for several days. The old yogi told him *"I feel pain but - there is no hurt in it"*.

Meares wrote that this let him know that you can use your mind to get the warning but the pain need not hurt. Months later, back in Melbourne, he had to have a tooth out. He asked his dentist to take this tooth out without anaesthetic. Reluctantly, the dentist agreed. Meares relaxed and, felt the dentist remove the tooth. Meares now knew that he could show people in pain how to do the same thing. Herbet Bower, another psychiatrist, wrote that Meares *"spoke increasingly about meditation... mysticism, self-hypnosis and control of body pain."* In 1967 Meares finished <u>Relief Without Drugs</u> which explains the relaxing mental exercise to reduce anxiety, tension and pain.

Stillness Meditation Period (~1970 On)

Ainslie Meares began to teach groups and continued to refine his method. He broadened its scope to include personal and spiritual growth. Stillness meditation was simpler and more sophisticated than the earlier method. Meares adapted the Zen Koan and wrote 11 poetry books during this period.

For more than a decade, Meares had a hunch that mental stillness could help more than reducing cancer pain. That it might influence the growth of cancer. Later on, Meares said that his colleagues had been most unhelpful and that he had underestimated the hostility. But as the number of people whose cancer was influenced by meditation increased the opposition lessened. Meares went on showing people how to meditate till he passed away in 1986.

Stillness Meditation has been referred to as natural mental rest. Getting enough mental rest is important but should not be at the expense of losing too much time to living. One meditates to live a better quality of life - a calm mind in a body at ease living an active life - that was Meares' vision. It was what he did himself.

A cancer patient tried to improve stillness by adding another method to it (ie without telling Meares what she was doing). She deteriorated. When he found out Meares was able to help her improve by simply being still again. This led him to categorise the types of meditation available in the West back then. Essentially, there were 4 categories. The first 3 are:
- thought based (eg mantras)
- sensory (eg visualisation)
- emotional (eg compassion) based meditation

In these 3 types, some combination of intellect & will, the senses and emotions are active.

In the **last category**, Stillness Meditation, there is little mental activity ie little or no thought, little or no sensation and little or no emotion as the mind becomes still – easier to understand after having been experienced.

Meares' term "Stillness" is now sometimes used by some whose meditation has little in common with Meares' method. Mantras, breathing, visualisation, emotion and so on are not Stillness. Stillness lies beyond mindfulness. Effortless. Awake - neither asleep nor unconscious. Clear - not drowsy. Simply still.

This little outline was summarised from the fully referenced biography in <u>Ainslie Meares on Meditation</u> that was compiled after searching libraries worldwide and reading everything that Meares' wrote (also see p45).

Non Fiction Books

A Better Life

Part 1 : To the Teacher
1. The importance of meditation
2. The teacher's image and self-preparation
3. The necessity for non-logical communication
4. Explanation, motivation and rapport
5. Getting started.
Part 2: To the Student
1. Common problems in a young person's life
2. A good experience of life?
3. Common physiological problems in young people
4. Starting to meditate
5. The meditation itself
6. How does meditation work?
7. What can you expect from meditation
8. Afterword, Bibliography   (1989; pages 140)

A System Of Medical Hypnosis

1. Nature of hypnosis (*suggestion, suggestibility, phenomena, communication with hypnotised patient, patient communicates with therapist, hysteroid aspects, theories of, atavistic hypothesis, atavistic hypothesis in relation to the phenomena*)
2. Induction of hypnosis (*motivation for hypnosis, emotional relationship, prestige, structuring the interview, choice of method, explaining hypnosis to patient, defences against, authoritative & passive approaches, moral & ethical aspects; induction by suggestion, arm levitation, repetitive movement, direct stare, dynamic method, other methods; waking, complications of induction, learning how to induce*)
3. Suggestive therapy (*principles & techniques; use with children; use in conditions & disorders [eg psychoneuroses, psychosomatic, personality, habit & psycho-sexual]; difficulties, complications, side effects, y state, case management*)
4. Hypnoanalysis (*principles & practice, regression in, abreaction in, special techniques, hypnography, hypnoplasty, dangers & complications*)
5. Hypnosis in general medicine (*insomnia, pain relief,*

anaesthesia, obstetrics & gynaecology, sundry uses, evaluation of place in medicine) (1960; 484 pages)

Dialogue With Youth
1. What is youth?
2. Youth and his idealism
3. Youth and his parents
4. Youth and his studies
5. Youth and society
6. Youth and his fellows
7. Youth and sex
8. Youth and his basic psychological drives
9. Youth and drugs
10. Youth and his search for identity
11. Postscript (1973; 288 pages)

Hypnography
1. Introduction – *historical background & origins.*
2. Preliminaries – *history taking, establishing rapport, prestige, assessing motivation, estimating suggestibility, explaining hypnosis to patient.*
3. Induction of hypnosis – *choice of method, by suggestion, by arm levitation, by induction of repetitive movement, the dynamic method.*
4. Description of hypnography – *technique, concluding the session.*
5. The paintings – *description, subject matter, emotional content, manner of production.*
6. The associations – *obtaining associations, nature of associations, emotional accompaniment.*
7. Psycho-dynamics of hypnography– *defences; meaning of behaviour, verbal & graphic expression.*
8. Symbolism in hypnography – *representation & conventional symbols, individual & universal symbols and evaluation of symbols.*
9. Excerpts from case histories – *cases 1-5.*
10. General considerations – *problems in technique, dangers of hypnography, sidelights on hypnosis.*
11. Assessment of hypnography–*in relation to therapy, hypnosis, symbolism & psych theory* (1957; 270 pages)

Let's Be Human

1. Changes in ourselves
2. Obsolete reactions
3. Anxiety and depression
4. Adverse reactions
5. Emergent reactions
6. Pleasure reactions
7. Education
8. Towards fully human reactions
9. Religion
10. Quality and purpose   (1976; 220 pages)

Life Without Stress

1. The nature of stress
2. Background problems
3. Major problem
4. Symptoms of stress
5. The background management of stress
6. Inferior ways of coping with stress
7. Stress and the quality of life
8. Meditation   (1987; 121 pages)

Management Of The Anxious Patient

1. The nature of anxiety- *introduction, recognising the anxious patient, simple theoretical considerations, failure of present day theories, atavistic theory of mental homeostasis, statement of atavistic theory.*
2. Common causes of anxiety- *nature of stress, susceptibility to anxiety, sexual causes, frustration of aggression, unsatisfied dependent needs, unconscious psychological causes, somatic causes of anxiety, spiritual conflicts.*
3. We talk with the patient- *nature of interview, rapport, communication with patient, elicitation of conflict, hostility, passivity, silence, physical examination, patient's anxiety during interview.*
4. Techniques for relief of anxiety- *explanation, reassurance, persuasion, suggestion, emotional support, abreaction, conditioning, hypnoidalization, drugs, environmental factors, psychotherapy.*
5. Special techniques- *free association, dream interpretation, painting and modelling, hypnosis.*
6. Nervous illness- *anxiety state, phobias, hysteria, obsessives,*

hypochondriasis, schizophrenia, melancholy, homosexual anxiety, immature personality, mentally retarded, habit formation.

7. Common syndromes with overt anxiety- *pain, alcoholism, childhood, the aged, iatrogenic anxiety.*
8. Some psychosomatic syndromes- *psychosomatic response, alimentary system, cardiovascular system, common psychosomatic disorders.* (1963; 493 pages)

Marriage And Personality

1. Extrovert personality
2. Introvert personality
3. Obsessive personality
4. Hysteroid personality
5. The paranoid personality
6. Psychopathic personality
7. The latent invert
8. Intelligence
9. Immature personality
10. Marriage, personality and alcoholism
11. Mature personality (1957; 157 pages)

Relief Without Drugs

1. Introduction
2. The nature of anxiety
3. Common causes of anxiety
4. Self management of anxiety [*via the relaxing mental exercise*]
5. Some notes about pain
6. Self management of pain
7. Conclusion, index (1967; pages 177)

Relief Without Drugs (RWD) is included in Ainslie Meares on Meditation (AMOM). RWD (in AMOM) includes the topics above. This includes the complete relaxing mental exercise and its application reducing tension and anxiety through to taking the hurt out of pain (also see p44).

Shapes Of Sanity

1. Introduction
2. Theoretical aspects of plastotherapy– *introduction, reduction of time, initiation & intensification of psycho-dynamics, emotional reaction.*

3. Technique of plastotherapy– *materials, explanation to patient, procedure with different personality types, rejection of modelling, precautions.*

4. Models– *general characteristics, meaning of models, previous experience in modelling, pseudo phallic symbols, screen models.*

5. Associations – *eliciting assoc., Manner assoc. Given, communication by non-verbal assoc., Defence by denial, nonspecific assoc., Defence by circumstantiality, emotional dissoc., Blocking.*

6. Psychodynamics of plastotherapy– *modelling as a catalyst, defence by camouflage, abreaction, patient's reaction, failed screens, second session resistance.*

7. Anxiety reactions– *in plastotherapy, from frustration, sudden awareness of repressed material.*

8. Interpretation of models– *means of interpretation, types of symbolism, levels of interpretation, reality problems, basic psychological conflicts, abstractions.*

9. Plastotherapy as an aid in diagnosis– *incipient psychosis, hallucinated hysteric, sophisticated psycho-neurotic, diagnosis of basic personality.*

10. Plastotherapy with psychotics– *modes of psychotics, modelling as communication, models act as a guide to progress, psychotic associations.*

11. Plastotherapy with psycho-neurotics– *models of psychoneurotics, the approach, gradual expression of conflict.*

12. Plastotherapy – *excerpts from case histories 1-5.*

13. Evaluating plastotherapy– *disadvantages, advantages.*

14. Hypnoplasty– intro. – *origin & purpose, type of patient.*

15. Guiding principles in hypnosis for hypnoplasty – *meaning of behaviour, dynamic concept of hypnosis, effect of patient's preconceived ideas, conditioning patient, motivation for hypnosis.*

16. Induction of hypnosis for hypnoplasty– *choice of method, arm levitation, initiation of repetitive movement, induction by dynamic method.*

17. Technique of hypnoplasty– *preliminaries, critical depth, initial suggestions, procedure in hypnoplasty.*

18. Models made in hypnoplasty– *description of models, specificity of models, plastic symbolism in hypnosis, relation to depth of hypnosis.*

19. Association to the hypnotic models– *eliciting associations, meaning of models, abreaction.*

20. Patient's defences in hypnoplasty– *nature of defences, defences against hypnosis, defences against modelling, defences against verbal associations.*

21. Psychodynamics of hypnoplasty– *ventilation of conflicts,*

emotional participation, modelling facilitates verbal expression, hypnoplasty affects state of hypnosis, toleration of conflict.
22. Anxiety reactions in hypnoplasty– *sudden awareness of hypnosis or repressed material, other causes.*
23. Hypnoplasty– *excerpts from case histories 1-4.*
24. Modelling as an adjuvant to psychiatric treatment– *occup, integrative, recreational & art therapy.* (1960; 450 pages)

Strange Places Simple Truths

1. Preface, Introduction, To those who travel
2. Burma, India, Nepal
3. Bali
4. Iran
5. Thailand
6. Mexico, Peru, Brazil
7. Mauritius
8. Africa - South Africa, Rhodesia, Kenya, Uganda
9. Ethiopia
10. Egypt
11. Russia
12. Taiwan, Japan, Korea, Hong Kong (1969; 225 pages)

A travel log of hypnotism, meditation & mysticism all over the world including Ainslie Meares meetings with yogis,witch doctors, healers, voodoo, copts, zen monks etc. The list of countries above have been grouped by area (eg Asia, Africa etc) for conveniance rather than replicating the structure of the book.

Student Problems & Guide To Study

1. The cause of lack of concentration
2. Things that make study difficult– and ways to meet them
3. Some basic problems
4. The bigger picture
5. Student life
6. Hints on study
7. Hints on exams
8. Mental exercises to reduce tension
9. Dangers in student life and study (1969; 108 pages)

The Hidden Powers Of Leadership

1. Identification
2. Imitation

3. Suggestion
4. Explanation
5. Logical communication
6. The ideas of our leadership
7. Gambits of leadership
8. The woman leader
9. Authoritative and passive leadership
10. Patterns of leadership
11. Why do people aspire to leadership?
12. The leader and the person we are
13. Ourselves as leader   (1978; 123 pages)

The Introvert

1. Introduction
2. The introvert child
3. Introversion in the girl
4. The adolescent introvert
5. Some aspects of introversion
6. Introvert's occupation
7. Introvert's leisure
8. Young adult introvert
9. The introvert and marriage
10. The introvert and parenthood
11. Outcome   (1958;142 pages)

The Door Of Serenity

Meares' case study on the therapeutic use of symbolic painting. The story of a young schizophrenic he helped come to terms with the traumas she had experienced. The book consists of the story and 24 paintings – one for each chapter.   (1958; 121 pages)

The Medical Interview

1. Motivation for interview - *in patient & physician*
2. Intellectual factors – *intro., patient assesses physician, eliciting significant conflict, patient assesses physician's reaction.*
3. Extra-verbal and non-verbal communication
4. Rapport– *nature of, establishing & obstacles to rapport.*
5. Passivity– *object of, pseudo & dynamic passivity.*
6. Hostility– *hostility in patient and in physician.*
7. Abreaction– *types, induction of, effects of.*
8. Suggestion in interview– *nature of, use of, counter-suggestion,*

persuasion.

9. Physical examination– *physical exam, psychological effects, symbolic significance, the physicians role.*
10. Silences– *nature of, defensive, meaning of, silence of serenity.*
11. Conclusion- *management of patient, basic difficulties, final assessment.* (1957; 117 pages)

The New Woman

1. What is the new woman?
2. The demand for equality
3. The desire for self determination
4. A changed concept of femininity
5. The influence of education
6. The effect of woman in the professions
7. Reactions to present day materialism
8. Thinking and acting in new ways
9. Changed patterns of psychological response
10. Seeking satisfaction in community life
11. New approaches to social issues
12. Reactions to sexology and pornography
13. A new type of marriage relationship
14. Sexual fulfilment
15. Effects of the new philosophy on children
16. The psychological reactions of parents
17. The new woman's inner life
18. The dangers of the new aspirations
19. Corresponding changes in man
20. Those who remain women of tradition
21. Fulfilling the new woman's personality
22. What of the future? (1974; 224 pages)

The Silver Years

1. The older phase- *don't spoil it, over reacting, wise man or fool, good life?, Miniskirt complex, dogooders, cargo cult.*
2. Stress and anxiety – *the truth about it, do you get irritated, scrutiny, the workaholic mum, damn!*
3. The value of change– *difficulty of change, using psychological defences, bee in bonnet & sacred cows.*
4. Personality and lifestyles – *women's libber in later life, retired workaholic, merry widow, hermit, grudges.*
5. Stress – *another look at it, coping with it, drugs, effects, background problems, man & woman, cancer.*

6. Quality of life– *what is it?, Understanding without logic, goodness, friendship & god, austerity & discipline of ease.*
7. Practical views– *when to retire?, widowhood, 2nd marriage, chicken!, my doctor, pamper yourself, vitality.*
8. Ourselves and others- *reassurance, changes in us all, the making of a fusspot, the ugly guest.*
9. The innermost me – *the innermost me, belief, making amends, locked away, do you pray?*
10. Doubts– *crossroads, what can we look forward to?, Starting again, good days and bad days, filling in time.*
11. Biologically, it's part of us- *happiness, are you a hoarder?, Lonesome, places revisited.*
12. Of man and woman– *what are they saying?, Man and woman, do you cuddle?, A new partner?*
13. Thoughts – *purposelessness, a good think, trivia and wider vision, priorities, never too late, truth or myth?*
14. Towards understanding– *time, celebrations, growing older & wiser, we see thing differently, a last fling.*

(1988; 231 pages)

This book is a collection of articles compiled into a book with some text added. Hence, some extra details are provided in italics. Also, refer p40 for first line index of 32 poems included in this book.

The Way Up (aka How To Be A Boss)

1. Your personality characteristics and how to use them
2. Coping with ourselves
3. Coping with others
4. Communication
5. Women on the way up
6. Obtaining information from others reluctant to give it
7. How to bring others to accept our ideas
8. Morale
9. Retirement
10. What is success?   (1970; 249 pages)

The Wealth Within

Part 1 - Mental Ataraxis
Summary & Introduction
1. The effects of mental ataraxis
2. The relaxation of the body
3. Experiencing the relaxation
4. The relaxation of the mind

Why Be Old?

Poetry Books

A Kind Of Believing

Belief,	.
I believe:	2
What we believe	3
Belief comes to us	4
Put your hand	5
Understanding comes to us	6
The child grows,	7
I listen for the whispers	8
Why think when thinking drives it away?	9
Write it down,	10
In the mist are shadows,	11
In the vastness	12
The vision splendid	13
Belief is a child	14
We try to deny it,	15
Slowly and silently,	16
It's all about	17
The bird builds his nest,	18
Its nice, its pretty;	19
Sift the grain from the chaff	20
That which we cannot see	21
Desire	22
Thoughts	23
Purpose	24
The stuff of life.	25
A tranquil mind	26
Let's live at ease	27
When we want something	28
You have thought	29
The perfume persists	30

17

Publication Date: 1984

A Way Of Doctoring

19

21

Publication Date: 1985

Cancer: Another Way?

Set free the healing!	91
With ulcers – OK,	92
Relaxed.	93
Relax, (how can I do it?)	94
Now listen,	95
Just the calm and the stillness,	96
Feel the healing!	97
Healing, (could you be more logical?)	98
Logical.	99
But tell me this.	100
Remember this. I	101
But surely!	102
If I don't *will* the growth to go,	103
Why do you make such a fuss?	104
Letting the healing all through us,	105
Is it our body that heals?	106
Cancer unfolds.	107
Death.	108
With cancer, (we need to understand.)	109
It's all in the depth,	110
It's simple.	111
Feel it.	112
I've nothing to lose,	113
Can you let yourself venture?	114
Is it worth it?	115
Those that come to see you.	116
If what you say is right,	117
Doctors are human beings	118
So you've got it.	119
With death, (the game is not for winning!)	120
You say, do this	121
Not again!	122
Why do you write in this style?	123
The purpose of all this	124
It's late,	125

Publication Date: 1977

Dialogue On Meditation

There's something more	1
If I were to come to you	2
I want to live,	3
Life is striving.	4
Is it really worth it?	5
I wish I could believe in it	6
You invite me	7
Something says	8
And who taught you?	9
I'm not a fool.	10
To be alert	11
It all seems so simple;	12
You don't really answer	13
I might as well tell you,	14
You say in doing this	15
Has it not occurred to you	16
I would seek	17
Is it not that meditation	18
From the way you speak	19
Meditate	20
I listen carefully	21
Why meditate, which seems so dull,	22
To be quiet and at ease	23
With all your talk	24
You seem to have	25
In life	26
Knowledge- (is that the secret?)	27
Scream at the children	28
You keep talking of something better.	29
All your talk	30
You keep on repeating the idea	31
Can you give strength	32
Can't you see	33
You talk,	34
I love her.	35

Your talk of meditation (confuses)	72
Sometimes, (you talk like a schizophrenic.)	73
I read what you write	74
I've found great joy	75
Like a dream out of nothingness,	76
They tell me	77
Those with cancer	78
You harp on the silence	79
Time hastens.	80
You talk of this other knowing,	81
Let's gauge your meditation	82
What should I feel	83
You speak (as if it were something beyond)	84
So many things;	85
I think I understand	86
Is it that you'd bring me (closer to God?)	87
I sometimes wish (I were closer to God.)	88
All about use is the unrest	89
I believe you claim too much.	90
One thing only (the fullness of love,)	91
Sometimes (I think your sayings)	92
What is meditation	93
Is meditation (akin to prayer?)	94
Old men like to talk	95
Is there something more	96

Publication Date: 1979

From The Quiet Place

There is no preface	..
Read this!	I
Why not reason it out?	2
What good will it do me?	3
I don't want the mystical	4
Of pleasure and happiness	5
How do we seek it?	6
Why have you come?	7

Help the healing	44
Help the healing	45
There's healing.	46
Why keep talking of stillness,	47
Feel the calm.	48
What should I do with my thoughts?	49
We let it come.	50
Do less?	51
We go deeply,	52
We go widely,	53
We go high?	54
How do we gauge it?	55
Build.	56
Let us grow.	57
Healing?	58
This is the end.	59
Let us examine it critically	60

Publication Date: 1976

How Distant The Stars

How Distant the Stars is mainly of historic interest. The poems date to a time during the earliest days of Ainslie Meares involvement in medical hypnosis up until 1949 - well before he had transitioned to meditation. Meares gave each poem a title. Both the title and first line are provided below. The first 5 poems make it clear that even back then he was experimenting with how poetry might be used in psychiatry. The poems are completely different from his later work. For those whose interest is reading poetry to help learn Stillness Meditation the later poetry books are recommended.

I. An Early Schizophrenic	Alone, I drift or life's wide sea,	1
II. The Melancholic	Statue of grief, he stares with distant gaze,	2
III. The Hypomaniac	Oh Doc, I feel so bright and gay,	3
IV. A Schizoid Episode	Are you a friend; believe me please,	5
V. A Dream	I float serenely though the air,	7
Jungle	Greenness stark that overpowers,	9
Sunbathing	Worship the Sun, my friend,	11
Drought	Across the plain the lonely line of posts	13

The Mountain	Lofty mountain, mighty power,	13
Jungle Stream	Why must I stand in silent thought,	16
Sunset	Shades are growing,	20

Publication Date: 1987

Let's Be At Ease

We toil for food and shelter.	1
Ease is a gift of nature.	2
Ease, (that state of mind,)	3
Ease explained	4
The ease that we seek	5
What power of man	6
We may call in our sleep,	7
Ease with our fellows,	8
Ease brings understanding	9
Ease (comes of communion with our fellows,)	10
At ease in all that comes to us,	11
Ease is the gate	12
Ease does not sit down	13
The things that we have to do	14
Ease, (the gift of nature.)	15
The key of life	16
Ease, (springs from our mind,)	17
Ease is not idleness.	18
Rest is not ease,	19
Who can escape a restless night	20
Ease is the mortar	21
Come, my dear,	22
How can I capture this thing	23
Many a way of loving,	24
Ease of quietness of mind	25
Ease is the rein	26
Ease (allows us to speak)	27
Ease, like love,	28
Alone and ease upon me;	29
The words of great men	30

Ease is born and ease begets	31
Without climbing the mountain	32
Who can separate cause from effect?	33
Ease is not drowsy.	34
Fun, games, banter,	35
In the wishing well of time	36
Storms lash the waters,	37
Ease is that incredible quality	38
Ease saves us	39
Ease is the touch of the loved one	40
What we have passes on by act of law	41
Coping is more than putting right	42
Ease (puts to flight)	43
There may come a sense of ease	44
The sun emerges	45
Ease (unties the leash)	46
There's a beginning for all.	47
Ease (the elusive one,)	48
The brightest star	49
Those who seek ease through meditation	50
When it is done,	51
Ease (frees us)	52
Ease, (Sunday afternoon,)	53
Disrobe,	54
The candle flickers	55
There may seem ease in death;	56
Our children, and so much to learn!	57
Ease (may come of a task well done.)	58
Like love	59
And the future,	60

Publication Date: 1987

Man And Woman

The moon	1
A woman	2
Woman is soft	3

33

The touch,	40
An arm around me.	41
Then comes the touch	42
Tender places	43
The wrappings of sleep.	44
The truth that comes,	45
Our soul,	46
With you,	47
My soul, (was estranged from me)	48
My soul, (I know you were always there)	49
Where am I going?	50
Think.	51
The dream of man and woman	52
Destiny!	53
It seems	54
Have you ever noticed	55
What have I learned	56
The wind blows your hair	57
I'm calling, calling.	58
I trust you in the simple things of life,	59
What does it mean,	60

Publication Date: 1987

My Soul And I

Nothing very much,	3
Teach me, my soul,	4
Out the door	5
As a child	6
To strive,	7
My soul,	8
Reason,	9
Invisible threads	10
It seemed good,	11
In my loneliness	12
Beyond the glassed pane at my side	13
It could be said	14

35

Publication Date: 1982

Prayer And Beyond

Publication Date: 1981

The Silver Years

Also see page 15 for synopses of **The Silver Years**

Thoughts

Publication Date: 1980

Miscellaneous Books

Meares' Audio, Braille, Translated Books

Audio Books - English

A kind Of Believing
Dialogue On Meditation
Cancer: Another Way?
Let's Be Human
Relief Without Drugs
Why Be Old?

Where Magic Lies
The Door Of Serenity
The Hidden Powers Of Leadership
The Introvert
The Wealth Within

Audio Books - Swedish

Bli Äldre Utan Att Bli Gammal *[Why Be Old?]*
Finn Ditt Inre Lugn. *[The Wealth Within]*
Avspänd Utan Mediciner *[Relief Without Drugs]*

Braille Books

The Wealth Within
Cancer: Another Way

Translated Books

Chinese
Cheng Gong De Ao Mi *[The Way Up]*
Dutch
Oud En Wijs *[Why Be Old]*
French
Un Psychiatre Chez Les Yogis Et Les Médecins Sorciers *[Strange Places Simple Truths]*
Soulagement Sans Drogues *[Relief Without Drugs]*
Korean
In'gan Kwan'gye Ŭi Ihae *[The Way Up]*
Italian
Rilassamento E Meditazione Con L'atarassia Mentale *[The Wealth Within]*
German
Ängstige Dich Nicht - Lebe Und Gewinne *[The Wealth Within]*
Japanese
Hito O Miru Me O Dō Yashinauka *[The Way Up]*
Jiritsu Kunrenhō *[Relief Without Drugs]*
Polish
Wycisz Strach [*In Stillness Conquer Fear*] by Pauline McKinnon

43

Russian
Podchiniat Eli Podchiniat Sia *[Hidden Powers of Leadership]*
Lechenie Bez Lekarstv *[Relief Without Drugs]*
Spanish
Los Poderes Ocultos Del Liderazgo *[Hidden Powers of Leadership]*
La Meditación Y La Relajación Como Tratamiento De La Inquietud
[The Wealth Within?]
Hipnosis Médica *[A System Of Medical Hypnosis]*
Swedish
Bli Äldre Utan Att Bli Gammal *[Why Be Old]*
Finn Ditt Inre Lugn *[The Wealth Within]*
Avspänd Utan Mediciner *[Relief Without Drugs]*

Books & CDs By Other Authors

Bruhn, Owen

Ainslie Meares on Meditation *(includes: Relief Without Drugs by Ainslie Meares, 30+ poems by Ainslie Meares; his later refined Stillness Meditation method, a biography of Meares' life and work, teaching protocol.* Also see p10*).*
A Key To The Books Of Ainslie Meares *(This book)*
Untitled *(In preparation: Meares' method integrated with evolutionary health)*

McKinnon, Pauline

In Stillness Conquer Fear *(Meares' method to overcome anxiety, panic & fear)*
Living Calm In A Busy World *(A guide to Meares' method)*
Help Yourself And Your Child To Happiness *(via natural stress management)*
Let's Be Still *(Manual: teaching stillness meditation to children & adolescents)*
Childrens Books:- Quiet Magic; Footprints In The Sand;
　　　　　　　　Joseph's Secret; Rainbow's End

Experiencing Stillness Meditation (CD) *(For adults)*
Natural Calm Meditation (CD) *(For those with prior experience)*
Let's Be Still *(CD) (For children & adolescents)*

Queensland Relaxation Centre Inc

Healing Power of Meditation *(CD) (Recording of a talk by Ainslie Meares)*

Reardon, Ray

Universal Reflections: Images of Relaxing Meditation
Relaxing Meditation. Theory & Practice (CD)

The End

www.ingramcontent.com/pod-product-compliance
Lightning Source LLC
Chambersburg PA
CBHW062153020426
42334CB00020B/2592